Diabetes

The Best Guide To Reverse Diabetes with 10 Proven Step by Step Strategies

Table of Contents

Introduction

Every journey begins with the first step. By purchasing this book you have already embarked on the journey to a healthier life, where only a little or no medications for diabetes will be needed. There is absolutely no need to worry. Even if you are 'diagnosed' to be at the borderline with diabetes, this guide will help you reverse the course and get back on the right track.

We all know that diabetes is a disease that can be controlled, but the truth is - it can also be reversed. No extra costs needed, no expensive 'cure' needs to be purchased. Just your strong will and determination are required in order to stop the havoc that diabetes has been wreaking on yours and your closest ones' lives. The only thing I ask of you is not to stray from this path and successful results are guaranteed. While reversing diabetes, this guide will also reward you with that fit shape you've always longed for, help you relax, provide you with your well-deserved beauty sleep and all with a giant smile on your face. Now, imagine that.

You doubt it's possible? Stuck at the crossroad of all the 'expert's' conflicting theories? Let this book be the navigator that will steer you in the right direction. Follow our 10 proven strategies and convince yourselves otherwise.

The rest of your life starts today

monetary loss due to the information herein, either directly or indirectly.

Respective authors own all copyrights not held by the publisher.

The information herein is offered for informational purposes solely, and is universal as so. The presentation of the information is without contract or any type of guarantee assurance.

The trademarks that are used are without any consent, and the publication of the trademark is without permission or backing by the trademark owner. All trademarks and brands within this book are for clarifying purposes only and are the owned by the owners themselves, not affiliated with this document.

Knowledge is Power

Many studies have shown that most people diagnosed with diabetes are actually ignorant about what is really happening in their bodies. It seems pretty impossible to fight off a disease if you are not fully aware of it, don't you think?

People don't say that knowledge is power for no reason. In this case, knowledge about this horrible life-threatening disease will give you the power to make permanent positive changes. Knowing what you're dealing with will make you accept these next steps more willingly in order to reverse or dodge diabetes.

What is diabetes? Unfortunately, diabetes is a chronic life-long condition where your body is incapable of using the amount of glucose properly, so it keeps piling up in your blood. How and why does it happen? To make it clearer, imagine fuel. Yes, fuel. Just like your car needs fuel to get from A to B, the same way your body needs fuel to perform every task, whether it's sleeping or running a marathon. Our body gets most of the fuel from the *glucose*. Once the food we've eaten is converted into glucose, it travels into our body (especially the liver and muscles) and brain, through our bloodstream. Glucose cannot enter our body cells without the hormone *insulin* that the pancreas produces. So when diabetes occurs and glucose is loaded in our blood, is due to the pancreas' inability to produce enough or any insulin.

There are two types of diabetes:

Type 1 Diabetes is a disease where the immune system attacks the healthy beta cells from the pancreas that produce insulin, because they are mistaken for bad invaders. This autoimmune condition causes damage to the pancreas that leads to cells' inability to create the required or in some cases any amount of insulin. This type is also called *juvenile* diabetes, because it mostly attacks young adults and children. It accounts for 5-10 % of the people diagnosed with diabetes. Although it is hard to reverse, the steps that this guide provide will help people with type 1 diabetes regulate their 'blood sugar' and feel much better overall.

Type 2 Diabetes is a condition where the cells are resistant to insulin. The body keeps up for some time by creating more than enough insulin, which will eventually lead to burned out receptors' sites. Because the cells do not accept the insulin any longer, the glucose cannot be transferred to the brain and body parts, and stays in the bloodstream. This is why the 'blood glucose' or as we call it 'blood sugar' levels are high. Type 2 occurs in 90% of the cases.

There are many people who are under attack by this disease, but are unaware that are diabetic. How to tell if you show signs of having diabetes? These are the most common symptoms that should ring an alarm that it's time for a medical checkup:

- Frequent urination

- Increased thirst

- Fatigue

- Unexplained weight loss

- Blurry vision

- Poor wound healing

- Extreme hunger

- Irritability

- Tingling in your feet and/or hands

For those of you who aren't diagnosed with diabetes and are reading this guide solely for educational purposes or are in pursuit of advice for someone close to you that is suffering from diabetes - it is critical that you also test yourself and determine whether you are really not confronting diabetes. It is crucial to do so, especially if you are affected by some of the diabetes' risk factors:

- You are overweight

- Have a close family member with diabetes

- Your HDL cholesterol is lower than 35 and your triglycerides level higher than 245

- Your blood pressure is higher than 140/90

- You are older than 45

- Your family background is African American, Hispanic American/Latino, Pacific Islander, Asian American or American Indian

- You had gestational diabetes during pregnancy

- Gave birth to a baby weighing more than 9 pounds

- You are physically inactive

However, even when you decide to test yourself, you should know exactly how to do it. Most doctors have been trained that when a patient wants to be tested for diabetes, they simply measure the glucose levels in their blood, 8 hours after their last meal. Do not get me wrong, this is a relevant test that clearly shows if someone has diabetes, it is just a poor indicator. Diabetes starts long before the *fasting glucose plasma test* confirms so. Now that we have explained how this horrible disease is created, you can only guess that the key to what has gone haywire is in fact the insulin. So, instead of measuring the 'sugar' in your blood, which is clearly not at the root of what has gone wrong, ask your doctor for an *insulin response test*. Do not wait for your doctor to diagnose you with diabetes and put you on medication if you have the chance to eradicate the process. If this test's results show high insulin, you WILL HAVE a chance to normalize it by following our next steps and stop diabetes from occurring.

Be Nutrition-Smart

It is scary. Receiving the news that you are affected by diabetes must definitely be one of the worst moments in your life. You know that it cannot be treated and you're labeled as diabetic for life. You have seen people struggle with this disease before and you must feel like the end of the world is coming. But it's not.

Although diabetes was known as irreversible for a long time, science has proven otherwise. You CAN reprogram your body so it can begin regulating the blood sugar again. Attacking this disease on the front of food consumption armed with properly balanced diet, you will force your body to repair the damage that diabetes has caused and make the glucose return to normal range, which will lead to its complete reversion. Your nutrition plays a major, if not the most important part when trying to fight off diabetes.

Resist the Temptation

Learning how to say NO to the juicy and delicious, but extremely unhealthy junk food is crucial for reversing diabetes. It's about time to fill your trash can with the fat-bombs lying around your house. You will also have to say goodbye to:

Sugar. When struggling with a blood sugar disease it is pretty clear that sugar is off limits. And when I say sugar, I do not mean just skipping the teaspoon in your tea or coffee cup; I also mean avoiding anything that contains refined sugar. Thinking about substituting it with raw honey? You might want to rethink this urge. Although honey or maple syrup might be slightly healthier versions - they still badly affect the glucose in your blood. Switch to stevia and say farewell to sweet food and beverages.

Grains. Wheat and other grains that contain gluten should be avoided at all times. They are packed with a huge amount of carbohydrates which can easily be broken into sugar only after a couple of minutes after they've been consumed. The intestinal inflammation that gluten causes, lead to glucose's spikes.

Conventional Cow's Milk. Dairy is amazing at balancing the sugar in your blood, but not if it comes from conventional cows. This is especially important for those who suffer from type 1 diabetes. The milk from conventional cows harms the body the same way that gluten does. Substitute it with sheep's or goat's milk and enjoy your favorite drink. Always purchase organic and raw milk.

Processed Food. Food loses most of its nutrients in the process of cooking, which can easily lead to inflammation, liver toxification and of course high levels of blood sugar. That being said, you should avoid processed and go for whole foods that will help you reverse diabetes.

You should also exclude dry fruit, soy, canola, packaged food, pretzels, butter and all kinds of frozen pre-cooked food from your diet.

Balance Your Diet

'What to eat now?' Besides the obvious 'why me' question, this must be the first thing that pops up into your mind on your way home from the doctor's office where you've been told the bad news. Living with this disease and being careful about the food you consume, doesn't need to make you feel deprived. Taking a healthy approach and making smart choices about nutrition doesn't have to be exhaustive. If you think that balancing your diet means eating boring and tasteless meals, you are so wrong. Once you get the hang of consuming healthy and properly balanced food, you can dig in to a variety of delightful dishes.

Make these superfoods your ultimate weapon in the kitchen and enjoy a challenging cooking that will reward you with reversed diabetes and improved overall health:

Green Vegetables are the most important food to focus on in order to reverse diabetes. Nutrient- dense, cruciferous, leafy greens and other green vegetables contribute to lower HbA1c (glycated hemoglobin) levels.

Non-Starchy Vegetables like eggplants, mushrooms, onions, peppers, garlic etc. are packed with phytochemicals and fiber and have effects on blood sugar that are almost nonexistent.

Nuts are a very beneficial superfood to diabetes, as well as our general health. Besides the fact that they contribute to losing weight, they also have inflammatory properties that prevent the resistance of insulin.

Seeds like chia seeds, pumpkin seeds, flaxseed etc. are rich in fiber and omega-3fatty acids and they lower the triglycerides and increase the good HDL cholesterol level which will help you reverse diabetes.

Legumes like lentils, chickpeas and beans are the perfect carbohydrate source. Due to their resistant starch, abundant fiber and moderate protein the release of glucose into your bloodstream can be significantly reduced.

Fruit like kiwi, berries, melon and oranges that are low in sugar will minimize glycemic effects. Rich in antioxidants and fiber, fresh fruits also contribute to reversing diabetes.

Vinegar decreases the glucose levels in your blood. A study has shown that two tablespoons of vinegar taken before each meal lowers your blood sugar for 25 %.

Besides these power foods, make sure to include fish that is high in omega 3-fatty acids, coconut and red palm oil, grass-fed beef and raw cheese to your diet.

Another healthy diet tips that will help you reverse diabetes:

- Make sure to include at least 1 ounce of fiber per day from high fiber foods that will slow down the glucose absorption.

- Sprinkle your cooked food with herbs like parsley and turmeric that will balance your blood sugar.

- Make a rainbow-colored selection of fruit and vegetables for each daily intake.

- Never skip breakfast. Missing the most important meal of the day will raise the glucose levels in your blood for the rest of the day.

- When you crave sugar, reach for some protein-packed food instead. A hard-boiled egg perhaps, is a perfect way to charge your batteries.

- Be creative. Make new and tropical salads with leafy greens, berries and citrus fruit and enjoy that zesty deliciousness while keeping your cells sensitive to insulin.

Their Majesties – The Supplements

Unfortunately, diabetes is a nutrition-draining disease. The elevated levels of glucose in your blood are programmed to cause substantial loss to most of the nutrients found in the urine which leads to deficiency of the vital water-soluble minerals and vitamins. I imagine you already got the hint that your well-balanced meals are not enough on their own. Since our body cannot perform our daily tasks properly without the sufficient nutrients, it is highly recommended for people with diabetes to take supplements that will replace all of the essential properties that the glucose kills, on daily basis.

When searching for the right supplements you will most likely come across many contradictory theories. Some say you need to spend tons of money on vitamin pills, while others state that the high-quality food is more than enough. Do not go fishing for the most convenient 'advice'. It is after all, your health we are talking about. No, you don't have to take a handful of pills before or after every meal, but you need to pay close attention that you're getting the right amount of nutrients that provide your body with the ability to properly use insulin.

The Definite Must-Haves

Some 'experts' in order to promote certain pills and load the pharmaceutical industry with tons and tons of helpless people's money may suggest, and even prescribe all kinds of "necessary" supplements for diabetes. Do not empty your wallet uninformed. Even though vitamins like b-complex, vitamin C, D and E must be in the center of each diet, there are no scientific studies that have proven these to contribute to diabetes' reversal. Besides, there is a huge possibility that the balanced diet you consume will provide you with those, without them being 'murdered' by your high blood sugar later. It is important that before you start taking supplements, educate yourself first. Below you will see the definite list of the supplements that has proven to promote reducing blood sugar:

1. **Alpha- Lipoic Acid** is a potent antioxidant, which is a substance that protects the cells from damage. ALA can be found in potatoes, liver, broccoli and spinach. It is proven that ALA decreases insulin resistance, lower glucose levels and reduces oxidative stress.

2. **Omega-3 Fatty Acids** are as we said, very important for reversing diabetes. They are found in fish like salmon,

sardines and trout and walnuts. If you do not eat fish, make sure to purchase omega-3 algal capsules. Studies have shown that it mainly reduces heart diseases, control glucose and lower triglycerides.

3. **Chromium** is the mineral that should definitely be an inevitable accompaniment on your journey to a healthy life with diabetes. It can be found in many foods (whole grains, meat, some fruits and vegetables etc), however, in very small amounts. That is why a capsule or a tablet of chromium chloride or chromium picolinate should be included in your diet.

4. **Magnesium** is of great significance for our body's capability to properly process glucose and it is also known for decreasing the insulin resistance. It can be found in many foods such as leafy greens, nuts and whole grains. According to one research, people who consume rich-in-magnesium food, have more than 15 % reduced risk of developing type 2 diabetes. Taking a magnesium supplement will help you keep your glucose levels in check.

Herbal Supplements

An increasing number of researches show that alternative natural medicine can reverse diabetes. There are many herbal supplements that can help you lower the blood sugar and promote a proper insulin production and usage. However, I highly suggest that before you start venturing down the store's aisles in search for this healthy additions to your diet, you have a word with your doctor first. Since he has probably put you on some medications, it is important that you consult with him first, as some herbal supplements may have side effects and can seriously interfere with your prescribed medications.

Read on for the most beneficial natural supplements:

1. **Cinnamon** is one of the cheapest supplements that can be found in every household. The extracts of this spice aid in a quick blood sugar's absorption. With only a half of teaspoon daily, you can significantly improve the glucose's levels.

2. **Bitter Melon** is a traditional Chinese medicine. Besides the fact that it relieves some of the most common symptoms in diabetes like fatigue and thirst, studies show that it also lower the blood sugar. Aim for 1/3 cup of bitter melon's juice a day.

3. **Fenugreek** has been used as a Middle Eastern medicine for thousands of years. It contains amino acids which are

known to up the insulin's release. These seeds have been also used in Indian cooking. Use it as a spice and reduce the high cholesterol and glucose in blood.

4. **Prickly Pear Cactus** is high in fiber and contains properties that are similar to those in the insulin. Although there are limited researches on this fruit's contribution to reversing diabetes, there are no known side effects, so it won't hurt to add it to your diet. If you plan on eating it as a fruit, consume ½ cooked cactus fruit per day. If it is unavailable in the supermarkets near you, check if the health food stores have it in powdered juice version.

5. **Curcumin** has proven to be very successful at reversing diabetes. Its beneficial compounds boost the glucose's control and promote prevention of this disease.

6. **Giniseng** has diabetes-fighting benefits that are used in the Asian medicine for generations. Studies have shown that ½ - 1 tsp of giniseng's tincture, three times a day, significantly slow the carbohydrate absorption and increase the pancreas' production of insulin.

7. **Green Tea** supports the body's ability to metabolize sugar. Besides, this magical beverage also lowers the risk for cancer and lowers existing bad cholesterol.

8. **Psyllium** can be found in common bulk laxatives and with only a 1/3 ounce a day, you can normalize the glucose in your blood.

9. **Bilberry** contains extremely helpful antioxidants in its leaves and fruit. This blueberry's relative can protect the nerves and eyes and may decrease blood sugar.

Remember to always seek medical opinion before purchasing any kind of supplement in addition to or instead of your medication.

Get Active!

In spite of the fact that it is mostly considered to be a hereditary disease, you will be surprised to know that physical inactivity has lately found its way amongst the top factors for diabetes' development. Being physically active on regular basis plays a key role in managing and reversing diabetes. In case you are wondering how they are linked so importantly, the secret lies in the muscles. Using and building your muscles while being physically active you train them to use glucose better; the fact that this way the insulin transfers the glucose into muscles and other body's cells properly, you also provide them with energy which will prevent high blood sugar.

It is never too late to get active. Even if you've been a couch potato your whole live, with your commitment to live a long and healthy life you can get rewarding results and reverse diabetes with our next tips.

Shrink Your 'Sugar Belly'

Do not get confused by the mixed messages from the Internet, magazines, people struggling with diabetes, friends or even health experts. Taking care of your weight has a huge impact on diabetes. Being such emerging pandemics, obesity and diabetes simply do not work well together. When combined, these life-threatening diseases will keep you on the passenger seat and take the shortcut for you, instead of allowing you to enjoy the long ride. It is time to take over and grab the wheel yourself. By managing your weight you will also manage your diabetes.

Although physical activity will help you shred pounds, it is important that you know which parts you should concentrate on first, and lose weight in the 'right' places. Before you grab your sneakers and dumbbells, work on your 'apple-shaped' figure first. If you keep carrying your pounds around your abdomen, instead of your thighs and hips, you are prone to more complications with diabetes. Stashing weight within your abdomen puts pressure on all of the abdominal organs and also liver. Therefore, your 'sugar belly' can be blamed for insulin resistance and loading your blood with gigantic amount of glucose.

Many researches have shown that measuring your waist size is much better predicator for this disease, than the body mass index. So, take a tape measure, place it around your abdomen (bare of course), exhale and measure. Women's waist must be under 35 and men's under 40 inches.

Bent-knee bench will help you trim your tummy. Lying on your back, put your legs in the air and bent your knees at angle of 90 degrees. Support your head, by placing your hands behind it. Tighten your abdominal muscles by lifting your head, neck and shoulders off the floor along with your rib cage.

Even if you think your busy daily schedules doesn't allow you to set aside the time for exercising (who doesn't), I strongly suggest you make the effort to find 30-60 minute activity period, because e after all, your health is at stake here.

Aerobic Exercises will help your body have enhanced insulin sensitivity and with that proper usage, your blood sugar will be significantly lowered, as well as the blood pressure, and it will also improve your bad cholesterol levels. This type of exercise will (besides reversing diabetes) also provide your health with benefits on so many different levels; it will strengthen your bones, improve circulation, relieve unnecessary stress and protect you from heart diseases.

However, even if it is ideal for people trying to lose weight and keep it off to find close to 1 hour for aerobic exercise every day, if you haven't been that active recently, you cannot just jump-start exercising at experts' pace. You need to start slow and gradually increase the time and intensity. I suggest you start with 5-10 minutes of aerobic exercise a day and increase your sessions by a couple of minutes each week. Overtime you will make sure about the improvement of your fitness, so you will decide how much more you're able to do. Remember to always start your exercise with moderate and then work your way up to vigorous intensity.

Here are some examples of aerobic exercises that have proven to contribute to reversing diabetes:

- Brisk walking

- Hiking

- Running/jogging

- Dancing

- Ice-skating and roller-skating

- Bicycling

- Rowing

- Playing tennis

- Swimming and other water aerobics

Strength Training (you may know it as resistance training) helps with lowering your glucose levels in the blood by promoting the proper insulin functions. It is also vital for building a strong bone and muscle structure which will reduce the risk for bone fractures and osteoporosis. Protecting muscle loss with this kind of training will help you burn more calories even when you rest. Isn't that something? Strength training will also provide you with an independent lifestyle throughout the years, which once you age well, you will be extremely grateful for.

It is recommended that you do a type of strength training 2 times a week, in addition to your aerobic exercises. Here are some examples of strength training that will help you lower your blood sugar:

- Lifting light weights

- Taking a strength training class

- Using resistance bands

- Exercises like pushups, lunges, squats and planks

- Any other activity that will build up your muscles

*According to a Canadian study people who did both strength training and aerobic exercises lost significantly more fat and dropped their percentage in the A1C (a test for blood-sugar levels) than those who just did one exercise.

Turn OFF the Stress

Diabetes and stress cannot coexist. The modern life today may be wrought with insecurities, hard situations and making difficult choices, but leading a stressful lifestyle can alter your blood glucose levels in so many ways. How many times have you found yourself worrying about even the least important things in your life? Trying to make your way through this disease and enjoy a long and healthy life, you simply cannot afford stressing over everything. Don't you think it's about time you learned how to deal with this urge? And here is how you can do it.

Have a Good Night Sleep

Diabetes and insufficient sleep usually go hand in hand. Not getting enough sleep causes increased release of *ghrelin* – the hormone that makes you want to eat and produces less *leptin* – the hormone that tells you when to stop eating. You can only understand how reaching for more food and breaking your balance diet can affect your blood sugar. The largest research on the link between diabetes and bad night's sleep has shown that insufficient sleep boosts insulin resistance by whole 82 % and raises morning blood glucose levels by 23 %.

Sleeping well through the night will help you release the stress and be refreshed and more relax that will also contribute to your diabetes-reversal plan.

Many diabetic people will tell you how they suffer from sleep-deprivation. But that doesn't have to be the case with you. If you find yourself tossing and turning in the middle of the night however, you might want to consider our few tips:

- Have a consistent sleep schedule and stick to it even if it is a weekend.

- Ban all the electronic devices from your bedroom.

- Keep your bedroom dark and cool.

- Exercises leave you feeling energized so be physical active earlier in the day.

Relax!

Although our modern society forces us to feel stressed about many things that life throws at us, when stress becomes chronic it can wear us down both physically and mentally. Combined with diabetes, stress can be an enormous health issue. Struggling to deal with your problems can lead to some serious complications associated with diabetes. We all deserve a break and if our health depends on it, we better work on finding our inner peace. There are many relaxation techniques that are beneficial to reversing diabetes. Meditation and yoga has proven to be the most successful ones.

Yoga. The number of diabetic people who are turning to some soothing yoga poses is increasing every day. The effect that this ancient Indian discipline has on reversing diabetes is undeniable. It rejuvenates pancreatic cells, promotes weight loss, exercises the muscles and keeps blood glucose in check. An Indian study performed on 123 people with diabetes who were practicing yoga, kept their blood sugar levels steady and also managed to lose a couple of pounds. There is no need to be the most flexible expert to take advantage of the benefits that yoga provides. Rent a DVD or purchase a book with Yoga poses and relax.

Meditation. Besides providing self-awareness this relaxing method will also help your body reduce its response to stress, slow the heart beat, lower blood pressure and most importantly lower blood sugar. Relaxing with meditation allows achieving *homeostasis* which is a body's balance and it has proven to be an effective component in treating diabetes. It doesn't matter if you decide to go with the transcendental or mindfulness meditation, relaxing this way will get you one step closer to reversing diabetes. Many books and CDs can help you master the art of meditating, so take a deep breath and say goodbye to stress.

Avoid Environmental Toxins

Breaking news! Companies manufacture approximately 3.25 billion tons of different chemicals every year. Breathing such polluted air into our lungs is very harmful,. An average person has 91 toxins in the body that cause immune dysregulation and inflammation. Being an autoimmune disease, you can guess how badly chemicals affect diabetes. They slow the metabolism down and interfere with the important body function of switching proteins to genes which induces insulin resistance and worsens the blood sugar. Sadly, the largely-created burden of toxins that surrounds us will only grow bigger over the years and there isn't exactly a way to permanently avoid the exposure (I highly doubt your plan is to keep your gas mask on at all times). You can however, reduce the risk and stop toxins from interfering with your diabetes reversal task. So what do you do?

Stay Away From Plastics

It may seem unbelievable to some of you but plastics are very much associated with diabetes. A group of chemicals found in many wide-ranging products like cosmetics, perfumes, building materials, clothing, toys, vinyl products and even medical supplies is linked with increasing blood sugar and this has been backed up by many studies. A Swedish research of 1000 older men has found that blood levels with the chemical *phthalates* double the risk of type 2 diabetes; Harvard scientists also performed similar studies on women and found out the same result. Another study examined the chemical BPA (found in many plastic containers and metal cans with food) in the urine and came with the result that those who had high levels of this chemical had a diabetes rate that was 50 % percent higher than those whose urine was with lower levels of BPA.

While these studies still haven't proven that those chemicals can cause diabetes, they all state that plastic chemicals can seriously disrupt the insulin production.

In order to reverse diabetes it is necessary to lower the risk of chemical-exposure as much as possible. You may not be able to entirely stay away from plastics but there is a way to avoid them. Always purchase phthalates and BPA free products. When buying plastic containers make sure they do not have the #3 symbol - it means the product contains PVC which is a plastic with additives.

What else can you do to prevent yourself from the risk of the toxins?

- Installing a water filter plays a major part in reversing diabetes in general

- Do not use personal grooming products and household chemicals if you do not really need them. Try to stick with the really necessary ones

- Switch to natural cleaning products

- Consult with your doctor and make a week-detox plan twice a year

- Go to the sauna

- Avoid artificial air-fresheners

- Skip products that contain a 'fragrance' ingredient

If possible, try to spend more time in the nature. The fresh air will not only keep you away from the industry chemicals, but it will also recharge your batteries which can be quite splendid, considering the fact that you are trying to reverse a chronic illness.

Say 'NO' to Your Bad Habits

Nobody is flawless. There are times when we all make some not-so-brilliant choices and are stuck to deal with the consequences later; whether we're talking about one-more-chocolate-cupcake-won't-kill-me kind of decision, or developing a serious health-concerning addiction. The choices we make and the habits we develop are part of who we are and some of them have a serious effect on our lives. Being accustomed to the things we do frequently is in our human nature, but so is having the willpower to do things differently. Just like anything else, once created, habits can be broken.

Living as a diagnosed diabetic it is of great importance for you to distinguish what habits of yours are beneficial to your fight with diabetes and what can leave an irremovable stain not only on this chronic disease, but on your overall health as well. Getting rid of your bad habits may seem like quite the struggle, but think about the positive outcome and how high your percentage for reversing diabetes will be. Besides, once you get used to living without these vices, it will be almost like they've never even been a part of your life, right?

Reconsider Having Another Drink

Luckily for all of the occasional-booze lovers, studies show that a moderate amount of alcohol is in fact beneficial for the health of diabetics as it may reduce the risk for heart diseases. So to all of you who were wondering, no, alcohol is not completely off limits when you suffer from diabetes. A research performed on women with type 2 diabetes has shown that those who consumed small amounts on alcohol decreased their risk for heart disease whereas those who abstained didn't. A similar study on people with type 2 diabetes and non-diabetic people who were consuming alcohol in moderation, has shown that only those who were diabetic lowered the heart-disease risk. If you were thinking about having a beer during the big game or a glass of wine at some party – you have a green light.

Still, you have to be careful and consume alcohol only in small amounts. It is ideal to **switch to water after the first drink**. If you want to reverse diabetes, you are allowed to say 'cheers' and that's about it. You should, however, consider all factors like special medications, so it is best to <u>seek your doctor's advice on how and when to consume alcohol.</u>

Also be aware that alcohol has the tendency to cause *hypoglycemia* (low blood sugar) which can cause dizziness, sleepiness and disorientation so you can easily be mistaken for being drunk.

These are the general tips regarding diabetes and alcohol:

- Avoid daily drinking. It is proven that one drink during the day blurs the vision.

- Always carry you diabetes ID necklace or bracelet if you are planning on having a drink.

- Drink only when your glucose levels are under control. Alcohol may sometimes lower your blood sugar, but it mustn't be consumed in addition to or instead of your medication.

- Consume alcohol only in combination with food.

- Do not drink on empty stomach.

- Never mix your drink with anything other than water and club soda.

- Sip slowly.

- Never drive for a couple of hours after having a drink.

Put Down Your Cigarette

You have heard it a million times before; you have seen it on cigarette packages, TV, read it almost everywhere – smoking is BAD for your health. But despite the red marks along the way, you are still walking on the same path, aware what this horrible habit does to your health. Combine smoking with diabetes and you'll create an unstoppable destroying force.

Do you know that smoking is three times more dangerous when you have diabetes? Are you really aware of the permanent consequences that this habit can leave on your health? Is it really worth the risk?

This health hazard can contribute to a numerous complications with diabetes. No matter what type of diabetes you suffer from, smoking can make it extremely difficult to control this disease and simply impossible to reverse it. Here is how unfriendly smoking is to your disease:

- Smoking elevates blood sugar levels.

- Diabetic smokers are 3 times more likely to die of cardiovascular disease.

- It damages your eyes. Being a diabetic you are at higher risk for glaucoma and cataracts which will eventually lead to diabetic retinopathy that may cause blindness.

- Increases the risk of kidney diseases.

- Promotes peripheral neuropathy which it means it damages the nerves of the legs and arms that cause poor coordination, pain and numbness.

- People who smoke and suffer from diabetes usually have poor blood flow in the legs which leads to ulcers, infections and may eventually lead to imputation.

Do you want me to go on or you've come to your senses and decided to put down your cigarette? If so, then get ready to quit. Have in mind that breaking this addiction can be nerve-wrecking so be prepared. There are different methods of quitting you can choose from, but many diabetics have stated that the 'cold turkey' (you simply stop smoking) might be the most suitable one. There are however, those who claim that quitting gradually will slowly 'kill' the need. Anyway, this is a whole different subject and it is up to your own personal preferences; the main point is to flush the cigarettes down the toilet. Seriously, having these remainders laying around your home it will make this process harder. Throw away your cigarettes, lighters, matches and ashtrays and fill your lungs with fresh air.

Take a Good Care of Yourself

Diabetes diagnosis is sadly a diagnosis for life. Your prescribed medications and other restrictions will become your life-partners, essential for your fight with this disease. It is undeniable that having to live with such illness that threatens your health on so many levels is super overwhelming. But being stuck with it doesn't mean you have no control over your own condition. As we've described in the past chapters - there are a lot of things you can do in order to improve your diabetes-situation.

Taking a good care of your wellbeing is crucial. Since diabetes attacks every organ in your body and have effect on even the tiniest blood vessels, being a diabetic you are at much greater risk of many infections and other health-conditions than the general population, and that is a fact you mustn't neglect.

If checking your condition is something you're used to overlook, get ready to change that today and get yourself on the right track to reverse this life-long disease.

Monitoring Glucose

Monitoring the glucose level in the blood is something a diabetic must do daily and in some cases even a couple of times each day. Checking your blood sugar is the only way to see how your disease responds to your medication and your lifestyle, and the only indicator that can show you if there is need for making changes.

How to do it? There are many different models for measuring blood glucose, but generally, they all work the same way – with a needle to prick your skin and strips that analyze the blood samples. You should refer to the user's manual of the model for instructions, although this is how it usually works:

1. Wash your hands.

2. Insert one strip into the meter.

3. Prick the side of your fingertip with your lancing device.

4. Touch the edge of the strip with your blood drop and hold until the results come.

5. Your blood sugar levels will appear on the display.

A result of 125 mg/dL or above means you have *hyperglycemia* (high blood sugar) and below 100 mg/dL indicates low blood sugar or *hypoglycemia.*

Monitoring your blood glucose at home doesn't replace your doctor's visits. Only he can advise you on the safe parameters for your special condition.

Medical Checkups

If you do not actively manage the onset of symptoms, diabetes can lead to serious long-term complications. Neither of the previously mentioned tips will help you succeed in reversing this disease, if you are not constantly aware of exactly what is going on in your body. Regular medical checkups are an inevitable part of proper diabetes care. Early detections on even the smallest infection can save you of a permanent health problem. There are some parts of your body that are most vulnerable to the diabetes' attack and as such they should have your utmost attention.

Eye Care

Since blurred vision is one of the symptoms of diabetes, you can only imagine how sensitive your eyes are when you are diabetic. Even though by managing your blood sugar you minimize your risk for eye problems like cataracts and glaucoma, as well as prevent blindness, it is extremely important that you see an eye care professional for a dilated examination at least once a year. Only your ophthalmologist can detect and treat retinopathy.

Besides the necessary annual checkup, see a specialist immediately if:

- You notice you have trouble reading.

- You have blurred vision.

- Your eyes have gotten red.

- You see spots.

- You feel pressure in one or both eyes.

- You see double.

Foot Care

People with diabetes are also very prone to having foot problems. That is why taking a good care of your feet is vital. Have your health care provider perform a complete inspection once a year.

Inspecting and caring for your feet yourself is also crucial. Here is how you do it:

- Look at your feet every day for cuts, red spots, blisters and swelling.

- Seek care if you have a foot injury or even an ingrown nail.

- Carefully wash your feet every day.

- Do not walk barefoot.

- Wear comfortable shoes.

- Protect your feet from cold and hot.

- Make sure your skin is soft and smooth.

- Always put your feet up when you have the chance. This will keep your blood from flowing to them.

Dental Care

When you are diabetic, your gums are more sensitive and so, the chances for oral infections are greater. A good dental care is required which includes regular dental visits, ideally every six months.

To stave off the problems, you need to:

- Brush your teeth twice a day.

- Choose a toothbrush that has soft bristles.

- Floss once a day.

- If you have dentures, remove and clean them every day. Never sleep with them on.

- Use a mouthwash without alcohol.

Skin Care

Do you know that every third person has a skin disorder caused by diabetes at some point in life? If they are caught early, most of these disorders can be prevented. See a dermatologist once a year to inspect your skin and advice you whether changes are in order.

Stick to these carefully selected tips and you are most likely to prevent skin problems:

- Always keep your skin dry and clean.

- Use talctum powder for places like groins and armpits.

- Avoid hot showers and baths.

- Your skin should be moisturized at all times.

- Do not use hygiene sprays.

- Use only mild shampoos.

- Treat cuts immediately.

- Keep your house more humid during cold months.

It is highly suggested that people suffering from diabetes monitor their blood pressure and cholesterol levels as well.

A Personal Approach

People are different. Just as one shoe size doesn't fit us all, one medication cannot cure all of us either. Some patients may react one way to a given treatment, some react differently and there are also patients that don't even respond to that particular treatment. Since doctors are unsure what treatment is best for a given patient, it is common to prescribe medications that helped the greatest number of patients first. But doesn't your time matter? Are you willing to experiment with medications and let your doctor shift you from one therapy to another in search for the most effective one? This was a wake-up-call for the American and European Diabetes Associations and time for taking some serious measurements without wasting the patients' precious time on ineffective therapies. The guidelines of their studies say that your blood glucose goals need to be based on your own personal risk factors. Although the number of other studies that back this one is more and more increasing, most of the physicians are still 'old school'.

When you are faced with such vexing condition as diabetes, and when your life is literally threatened, you are the one who should pull the strings. You shouldn't avoid the guidelines of those studies. In fact, you should use them as you jumping-off point and tell your doctor that you want to find the suitable treatment with the _personalized medicine_ - *an emerging concept that treats patients with therapy that is determined on specific individual information.* It is recommended that diabetics as individuals decide with their doctors on what blood sugar target suits their needs the best, considering the four main personal-centered factors:

1. Identification of the biomarkers and genes for diabetes.

2. Allocating the resources to prevent/detect diabetes.

3. Selecting an individualized therapy, prescribing medication.

4. Measuring the circulating biomarkers in order to monitor the response to given treatment.

Many diabetics have found the patient-centered treatment a breath of fresh air. This kind of therapy is most likely to be the most beneficial for you and be the fuel that will keep you going on your journey to reversing diabetes.

We can only hope that the day when the personalized medicine will become the main theme of all the health guidelines is just around the corner.

Stay Strong Emotionally

Shock – is what usually people feel when they first hear the tragic news that they're under diabetes' attack. So many things change. Early diagnosed diabetics say that the unexpected niceness of people, the awkward situations, as well as the skills to maneuver them positively while trying to stay strong, wear them out. Besides socially, this disease has yet another way to keep you down. The level of progressiveness of the diabetes is high enough to require a lot of patient involvement. So many doctor's visits, numerous tests, sudden restrictions and lifestyle changes can have a bad effect on you, not only psychically, but also physically. Getting out of the house might turn into a physical challenge and spending time with your friend into a torture. Even though every diabetic has been through the not-in-the-mood-for-anything phase, learning to cope with this illness as better as you can is the only way you can be one step ahead of it and eventually reverse it.

You Are Not Alone

Seek for emotional support. You may be tough as a rock, but at fragile times like fighting a disease, everyone needs to 'hold someone's hand'. Assemble you own 'support team' that will help you through the challenging task of reversing diabetes. A study of the University of Pittsburgh has shown that those patients that teamed up with their doctors or family members increased their success of managing to hit healthy blood glucose and cholesterol levels by more than 40 %.

Remember than you are not alone. Over 29 million Americans suffer from diabetes. There are many support groups, forums and chat rooms online. Sign up to some of them. Sharing your personal story with people who are walking in your shoes will boost your confidence and help you not to stray from your balanced lifestyle for reversing diabetes.

Many people say that keeping a diary has also helped them stay strong emotionally. Try writing down how you feel on days when you're struggling to fake a smile; just as long tomorrow you'll be you're old self. Be careful not to give into depression, as it is common for diabetes and depression to occur together. If you find yourself showing signs of depression (sleeping more than usual or not getting any sleep, being sad for no reason, lacking interest in things you love doing, change in your eating habits etc.) talk to your doctor. Do not let depression go undiagnosed. He will help you to find the right treatment that will help you stick with your reversing-diabetes plan.

Conclusion

Now that you have learned what you have to do in order to reverse diabetes, the final tip I would like to provide you with is to START ACTING TODAY. Only if you take control over diabetes and not the other way around, you can enjoy life to the fullest, as if you were never even diagnosed.

These 10 tips have changed the lives of many diabetics for better, and they can do the same to you. Take the advantage of the content of this book and use it as a secret weapon in your battle with diabetes. I guarantee results so successful, you'll have to pinch yourself to make sure you're not dreaming. Sounds unbelievable? I dare you to try to show me otherwise.

With this guide, healthy life is indeed within reach.

BEFORE YOU GO

If you liked this book you may like these other books from Lee Douglas

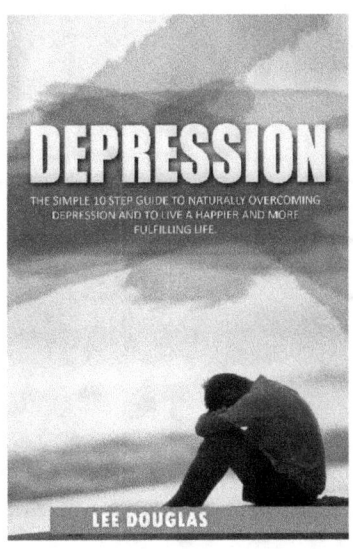

>>Check out more books by Lee Douglas<<

Free Gift

As Promised Here Is Your Guide To Managing Stress: Discover The Simple Solutions to Live A Stress Free Life.

GET YOUR COPY HERE

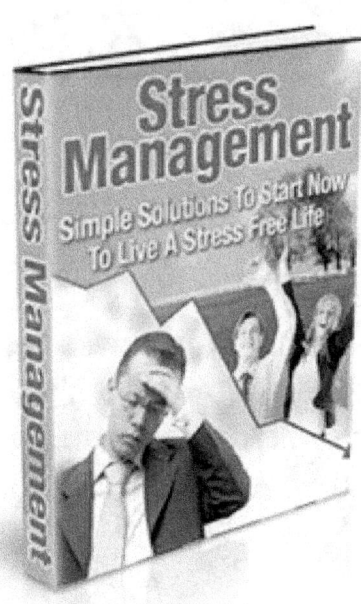

LEARN HOW TO MANAGE YOUR STRESS

Stress can take a huge chunk of your time, energy, and health. Not only your personal relationships suffer, but so as your career and total wellness. Are you struggling from stress? This book explains the true definition of stress, the symptoms and the right way to cure it. Moreover, the book gives tactical strategies to decrease your stress and increase living a happier and healthier life.

If You Want Free Best Selling Kindle Books Delivered Straight To Your Inbox

JOIN OUR FREE KINDLE BOOK CLUB!

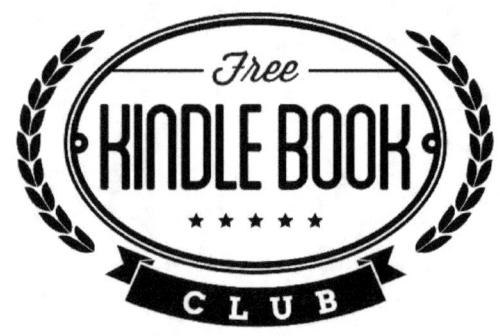

CLICK HERE

Finally, if you enjoyed this book, then I'd like to ask you for a favor, would you be kind enough to leave a review for this book on Amazon? It'd be greatly appreciated!

Thank you and good luck! ☺